Menopause

By

Dr. Steve J. Hayes

Table Of Contents

Introduction

Menopause is a moment a year after a lady's last period. The years paving the way to that point, when ladies might have changes in their month to month cycles, hot glimmers, or different side effects, are known as the menopausal progress or perimenopause. The menopausal progress most frequently starts between ages 45 and 55.

Chapter 1

Menopause

Menopause is a moment when an individual has gone 12 successive months without a feminine period. Menopause is a characteristic piece of maturing and denotes the finish of your conceptive years. By and large, menopause occurs at age 51.

What is menopause?

Menopause is a particular moment when you've gone 12 sequential months without a period. The time paving the way to menopause is called perimenopause. This is the point at which a lot of ladies or individuals relegated females upon entering the world (AFAB) begin to progress to menopause. They might see changes in their feminine cycles or have side effects like hot blazes.

What are the three phases of menopause?

Regular menopause is the long-lasting completion of the feminine cycle that doesn't occur as a result of clinical treatment. The cycle is slow and occurs in three phases:

Perimenopause or "menopause progress": Perimenopause can start eight to 10 years before menopause when your ovaries steadily produce less estrogen. It typically begins when you're in your 40s. Perimenopause endures up until menopause, the moment that your ovaries quit delivering eggs. In the final remaining one to two years of perimenopause, the drop in estrogen speeds up. At this stage, many individuals might encounter menopause side effects. Yet, you're actually having periods during this time and can get pregnant.

- **Menopause:** Menopause is the moment that you never again have feminine periods. At this stage, your ovaries have quit delivering eggs and quit creating the greater part of their estrogen. A medical services supplier analyzes menopause when you've done without a feminine period for 12 continuous months.

- **Postmenopause:** This is the name given to the time after you haven't had a period for a whole year (or the remainder of your life after menopause). During this stage, menopausal side effects, like hot glimmers, may improve. In any case, certain individuals keep on encountering menopausal side effects for 10 years or longer after the menopause change. Because of a lower estrogen level, individuals in the postmenopausal stage are at an expanded gamble for a few medical issues, like osteoporosis and coronary illness.

What is the ordinary age for menopause?

The typical time of menopause in the US is around 51 years of age. Nonetheless, the progress to menopause normally starts in your mid-40s.

Side effects And Causes

What are the indications of menopause?

You might be progressing into menopause assuming you start encountering some or the accompanying side effects as a whole:

- Hot blazes, otherwise called vasomotor side effects (an unexpected sensation of warmth that spreads over your body).
- Night sweats or potentially cool blazes.
- Vaginal dryness causes uneasiness during sex.
- Urinary direness (a squeezing need to pee all the more as often as possible).
- Trouble resting (a sleeping disorder).
- Profound changes (peevishness, temperament swings, or gentle wretchedness).
- Dry skin, dry eyes, or dry mouth.
- Bosom delicacy.
- Deteriorating premenstrual condition (PMS).
- Unpredictable periods or periods that are heavier or lighter than expected.
- Certain individuals could likewise insight:
- Dashing heart.
- Cerebral pains.
- Joint and muscle throbbing painfulness.

- Changes in moxie (sex drive).
- Trouble concentrating or memory slips (frequently impermanent).

- Weight gain.
- Going bald or diminishing.

Changes in your chemical levels cause these side effects. Certain individuals might have serious side effects of menopause, while others have gentle side effects. Not every person will have similar side effects as they progress to menopause.

Contact a medical services supplier on the off chance that you're uncertain assuming your side effects are connected with menopause or another medical issue.

How long do you have side effects of menopause?

You can have side effects of menopause for as long as 10 years. In any case, a great many people experience side effects of menopause for under five years.

What are hot glimmers and how long will I have them?

Hot glimmers are one of the most successive side effects of menopause. It's a concise vibe of intensitBesideside the intensity, hot glimmers can likewise accompany:

- A red, flushed face.
- Perspiring.
- A chilled feeling after the intensity.

The power, recurrence, and length of hot blazes vary for every person. Commonly, hot glimmers are less serious over the long haul.

For what reason does menopause occur?

At the point when menopause occurs all alone (regular menopause), it's a typical piece of maturing. Menopause is characterized as a total year without feminine dying, without medical procedure or ailment that might make ke draining stop, for example, hormonal contraception, radiation treatment, or careful expulsion of your ovaries.

As you age, your regenerative cycle starts to dial back and gets ready to stop. This cycle has been persistently working since pubescence. As menopause approaches,

your ovaries make to a lesser extent a chemical called estrogen. At the point when this lessening happens, your monthly cycle (period) begins to change. It can become sporadic and afterward stop.

Actual changes can likewise occur as your body adjusts to various degrees of chemicals. The side effects you experience during each phase of menopause (perimenopause, menopause, and postmenopause) are essential for your body's acclimation to these changes.

What hormonal changes occur during menopause?

The customary changes we consider "menopause" happens when your ovaries never again produce elevated degrees of chemicals. Your ovaries are the regenerative organs that store and deliver eggs. They additionally produce the synthetic compounds estrogen and progesterone. Together, estrogen and progesterone control the period. Estrogen additionally impacts how your body utilizes calcium and keeps up with cholesterol levels in your blood.

As menopause approaches, your ovaries never again discharge eggs, and you'll triumph ultimately over your last period.

How can I say whether I'm in menopause?

You'll realize you've arrived at menopause when you've gone 12 back-to-back a very long time without a feminine period. Contact your medical services supplier assuming that you have any sort of vaginal draining after menopause. Vaginal draining after menopause could be an indication of a more serious medical problem.

Determination And Tests

How is menopause analyzed?

There are multiple ways your medical services supplier can analyze menopause. The first is talking about your monthly cycle throughout the past year. Menopause is exceptional in that your supplier analyzes a large number of its happens. On the off chance that you've gone an entire year (12 straight months) without a period, you've entered menopause and might be postmenopausal.

The executives And Treatments

Might menopause at any point be dealt with?

Menopause is a characteristic cycle that your body goes through. Now and again, you may not require any treatment for menopause. While examining treatment for menopause with your supplier, about treating the side effects of menopause disturb your life. There are a wide range of kinds of medicines for the side effects of menopause. The fundamental kinds of treatment for menopause are:

- Chemical treatment.
- Nonhormonal medicines.

It's critical to converse with your medical services supplier while you're going through menopause to create a therapy plan that works for you. Each individual is unique and has one-of-a-kind necessities.

How is a chemical treatment for menopause?

During menopause, your body goes through major hormonal changes — diminishing how much chemicals it makes. Your ovaries produce estrogen and progesterone. At the point when your ovaries never again make sufficient estrogen and progesterone, chemical treatment can compensate for lost chemicals. Chemical treatment supports your chemical levels and can assist with side effects preferring hot blazes and vaginal dryness. It can likewise assist with forestalling osteoporosis.

There are two principal sorts of chemical treatment:

Estrogen treatment (ET): In this treatment, you take estrogen alone. Your supplier recommends it in a low portion. Estrogen comes in many structures, like a fix, pill, cream, vaginal ring, gel, or splash. Estrogen treatment is definitely not a decent treatment for you in the event that you actually have a uterus.

Estrogen Progesterone/Progestin Chemical Treatment (EPT): This treatment is likewise called mix treatment since it utilizes dosages of estrogen and progesterone. Progesterone is accessible in its normal structure, or likewise as a progestin (a manufactured type of progesterone). This kind of chemical treatment is for individuals who actually have their uterus.

Are there any dangers to chemical treatment?

The well-being dangers of chemical treatment include:

Endometrial malignant growth (possibly expanded assuming you use estrogen treatment regardless have your uterus).

- Gallstones and gallbladder issues.
- Blood clusters.
- Profound vein apoplexy.
- Aspiratory embolism.
- Stroke.

These dangers are lower on the off chance that you start chemical treatment in something like 10 years of menopause. After that point, your gamble for cardiovascular sicknesses is higher.

A relationship exists between extreme hot blazes and night sweats and your gamble for cardiovascular infection. Medical services suppliers might recommend beginning chemical treatment assuming you have these serious side effects since it's a marker for future cardiovascular gambling.

Going on chemical treatment is an individualized choice. Examine all previous ailments and your family ancestry with your medical services supplier to comprehend the dangers versus advantages of chemical treatment.

What are nonhormonal medicines for menopause?

However chemical treatment is an extremely viable technique for easing menopause side effects, but it's not the ideal treatment for everybody. Nonhormonal medicines incorporate changes to your eating regimen and way of life. These therapies are much of the time great choices for individuals who have other ailments or have as of late been treated for bosom disease. The primary non-hormonal medicines that your supplier might suggest include:

- Changing your eating routine.
- Keeping away from triggers to hot glimmers.

- Working out.
- Joining support gatherings.
- The doctor prescribed meds.

Diet

Some of the time changing your eating regimen can assist with alleviating menopause side effects. Restricting how much caffeine you eat consistently and scaling back hot food varieties can make your hot glimmers less serious. You can likewise add food sources that contain plant estrogen into your eating regimen. Plant estrogen (isoflavones) isn't a trade for the estrogen your body makes before menopause. Food sources to attempt include:

- Soybeans.
- Chickpeas.
- Lentils.
- Flaxseed.
- Grains.
- Beans.
- Natural products.

Vegetables.

Keeping away from triggers to hot blazes

Certain things in your day-to-day existence could be triggers for hot blazes. To assist with easing your side effects, attempt and distinguish these triggers and work around them. This could incorporate keeping your room cool around evening time, wearing layers of apparel, or Quitting smoking. Weight reduction can likewise assist with hot blazes.

Working out

Working out can be troublesome assuming that you're managing hot glimmers, yet practicing can assist with freeing a few different side effects from menopause. Exercise can assist you with staying asleep from sundown to sunset and is suggested on the off chance that you have sleep deprivation. Quiet, peaceful sorts of activity like yoga can likewise assist with your temperament and ease any apprehensions or nervousness you might feel.

Joining support gatherings

Conversing with others who are likewise going through menopause can be an incredible help for some. Joining a care group can not just give you a source for the numerous feelings going through your mind, yet additionally assist you with responding to questions you may not actually realize you have.

Doctor prescribed meds

Doctor-prescribed meds like estrogen treatment (estrogen in a cream, gel, or pill), contraception pills, and antidepressants (SSRIs and SNRIs) can assist with overseeing side effects of menopause like emotional episodes and hot blazes. Remedy vaginal creams can assist with easing vaginal dryness. A seizure medicine called gabapentin has been displayed to ease hot blazes. Talk with your medical services supplier to check whether nonhormonal prescriptions could work for dealing with your side effects.

Viewpoint/Forecast

Might I at any point get pregnant during menopause?

The chance of pregnancy vanishes once you're postmenopausal. Be that as it may, you can get pregnant during the menopause change (perimenopause). To become pregnant, you ought to keep on utilizing some type of conception prevention until you're certain you've gone through menopause. Ask your medical services supplier before you quit utilizing contraception.

What are the drawn-out well-being gambles related to menopause?

There are a few circumstances that you could be at a higher gamble of after menopause. Your gamble for any condition relies upon numerous things like your family ancestry, your well-being before menopause, and your way of life factors. Two circumstances that influence your well-being after menopause are osteoporosis and coronary supply route illness.

Osteoporosis

Osteoporosis, a "weak bone" infection, happens when the internal parts of bones become less thick, making them more delicate and liable to crack. Estrogen assumes a significant part in saving bone mass. Estrogen signals cells during the issues that remain to be worked out separating.

People lose a typical of 25% of their bone mass from the hour of menopause to develop 60. This is to a great extent a result of the deficiency of estrogen. Over the long run, this deficiency of bone can prompt bone breaks. Your medical care supplier might need to test the strength of your bones over the long haul. Bone mineral thickness testing, likewise called bone densitometry, is a speedy method for perceiving the amount of calcium you possess in specific pieces of your bones. The test is utilized to recognize osteoporosis and osteopenia. Osteopenia is an illness where bone thickness is diminished and this can be a forerunner to later osteoporosis.

Assuming that you have osteoporosis or osteopenia, your treatment choices could incorporate estrogen treatment.

Coronary corridor infection

Coronary corridor infection is the restricting or blockage of courses that supply your heart muscle with blood. This happens when greasy plaque develops in the corridor walls (known as atherosclerosis). This development is related to elevated degrees of cholesterol in your blood. After menopause, your gamble for coronary conduit infection builds in light of a few things, including:

- The deficiency of estrogen.
- Expanded circulatory strain.
- A diminishing in actual work.

A certain way of life propensities from your past finding you (like smoking or exorbitant liquor utilization).

Will chemical treatment assist with forestalling long-haul well-being gambles?

The advantages and dangers of chemical treatment fluctuate contingent upon your age and well-being history. As a general rule, more youthful individuals in their 50s will quite often seek additional advantages from chemical treatment contrasted with the people who are postmenopausal in their 60s. Individuals who go through untimely menopause frequently get chemical treatment until age 50 to compensate for the additional long periods of estrogen misfortune.

Living With

Could menopause at any point influence rest?

Certain individuals might encounter inconvenience staying asleep for the entire evening and sleep deprivation during menopause. This can be a typical result of menopause itself, or it very well may be because of one more side effect of menopause. Hot blazes are a typical guilty party of restless evenings during menopause.

Could menopause at any point influence my sexual coexistence?

After menopause, your body has less estrogen. This significant change in your hormonal equilibrium can influence your sexual coexistence. Many individuals encountering menopause might see that they're not quite so handily excited as in the past. Once in a while, individuals likewise might be less delicate to contact and other actual contact than before menopause.

These sentiments, combined with the other profound changes you might be encountering, can all prompt a diminished interest in sex. Remember that your body is going through a great deal of progress during menopause. A portion of different variables that can assume a part in a diminished sex drive can include:

- Having bladder control issues.
- Experiencing difficulty staying asleep for the entire evening.
- Encountering pressure, nervousness, or sorrow.
- Adapting to other ailments and drugs.

These variables can upset your life and even reason strain in your relationship(s). Notwithstanding these changes, the lower levels of estrogen in your body can cause a decline in the blood supply to your vagina. This can cause dryness. At the point when you don't have the perfect proportion of oil in your vagina, it can prompt difficult intercourse.

Feel free to converse with your medical services supplier about any declines you're encountering in your sex drive. Your supplier will talk about choices to assist you with feeling improved. For instance, you can treat vaginal dryness with over-the-counter (OTC), water-dissolvable, or silicone greases. Your medical care supplier can likewise recommend estrogen or non-estrogen chemicals to treat the vaginal tissue. They can endorse this in a low-portion cream, pill, or vaginal ring.

Do all menopausal individuals encounter a lessening in sexual craving?

Not all individuals experience diminished sexual longing. Now and again, it's the exact inverse. This could be on the grounds that there could be as of now not any apprehension about getting pregnant. For some, this permits them to appreciate sex without stressing over family arrangements.

Be that as it may, it's as yet essential to utilize security (condoms) during sex in the event that you're not in a monogamous relationship. You actually need to safeguard yourself from physically sent diseases (STIs). You can get an STI whenever in your life, even after menopause.

Could I at any point get pregnant assuming I've gone through menopause?

No, you can't get pregnant after menopause since ovulation is done happening.

Regularly Clarified some things

Does menopause cause weight gain?

It might. Chemical changes can affect your weight. For instance, you might begin to lose muscle as you age, which can influence how your body puts on weight.

Does menopause influence your teeth or mouth?

Indeed. Your teeth and gums are powerless against the hormonal changes that happen during menopause. This can prompt observable side effects like a dry mouth or touchy teeth and gums. This could build your gamble of creating holes or gum disease.

Does menopause influence your eyes?

Indeed. One of the side effects of the change to menopause is dry eyes.

Could menopause at any point cause beard growth development?

Indeed, beard growth development can be a change connected with menopause. This is on the grounds that testosterone is moderately higher than estrogen. On the off chance that your beard turns into an issue for you, waxing or utilizing other hair removers might be a choice.

Is struggling with concentrating and being careless an ordinary piece of menopause?

Tragically, focus and minor memory issues can be a typical piece of menopause. However this doesn't occur to everybody, it can work out. Assuming you're having memory issues during menopause, call your medical services supplier. A few exercises have been displayed to invigorate the mind and assist with reviving your memory. These exercises can include:

- Doing crossword puzzles and other intellectually invigorating exercises like perusing and doing numerical statements.
- Scaling back casual exercises like sitting in front of the television.
- Getting a lot of activity.
-

What is untimely menopause?

Menopause, when it happens between the ages of 45 and 55, is thought of as "regular" and is an ordinary piece of maturing. Menopause that happens before the age of 45 is called early menopause. Menopause that happens at 40 or more youthful is viewed as untimely menopause. At the point when there's no

clinical or careful reason for untimely menopause, it's called essential ovarian inadequacy.

Could menopause at any point cause misery?

Indeed, a few elements connected with menopause can prompt wretchedness. Your body goes through a great deal of changes during menopause. There are outrageous changes in your chemical levels, you may not rest soundly on account of hot glimmers and you might encounter state of mind swings. Nervousness and dread could likewise be affecting everything during this time.

Assuming you experience any of the side effects of discouragement, converse with your medical care supplier. During your discussion, your supplier will inform you regarding various sorts of therapy and check to ensure there is no other ailment causing your downturn.

Are there other profound changes that can occur during menopause?

Menopause can cause various close-to-home changes, including:

- An absence of inspiration and trouble concentrating.
-

- Uneasiness, sadness, state of mind changes, and strain.
- Forcefulness and peevishness.

These close-to-home changes can occur beyond menopause, as well. You've most likely encountered some of them all through your life.

Your medical care supplier might have the option to recommend a prescription to help you (chemical treatment or an energizer). It might likewise serve to simply realize that there's a name for the sentiments you're encountering. Support gatherings and guidance are valuable apparatuses while managing close-to-home changes during menopause.

How does menopause influence my bladder control?

Sadly, bladder control issues (likewise called urinary incontinence) are normal for individuals going through menopause. There are a few motivations behind why this occurs, including:

Estrogen. Estrogen assumes many parts in your body, including keeping the coating of your bladder and urethra solid.

Pelvic floor muscles. They support the organs in your pelvis — your bladder and uterus. All through your life, these muscles can debilitate. This can occur during pregnancy, labor, and from weight gain. At the point when the muscles debilitate, you can encounter urinary incontinence (spillage).

Will I start menopause on the off chance that I have a hysterectomy?

It relies upon assuming that your specialist likewise eliminated your ovaries during the hysterectomy. Assuming you kept your ovaries, you might not have side effects of menopause immediately. On the off chance that your specialist additionally eliminates your ovaries, you'll have side effects of menopause right away.

Might I at any point have a climax after menopause?

Indeed, you can in any case have a climax after menopause. A climax might feel hard to accomplish whenever you've arrived at menopause, yet there's no great explanation to keep you from having a climax.

Do men go through menopause?

Andropause, or male menopause, is a term that portrays diminishing testosterone levels in men or individuals doled out male upon entering the world (AMAB). Testosterone creation in men declines around 1% each year — significantly more slowly than estrogen creation in ladies. Medical services suppliers frequently banter calling this sluggish decrease in testosterone "menopause" since it's not as extreme of a chemical shift and doesn't convey similar power of secondary effects as menopause in ladies. A few men won't see the change since it occurs over numerous years or many years. Different names for the male rendition of menopause are age-related low testosterone, male hypogonadism, or androgen inadequacy.

Note

Menopause is a characteristic and typical piece of the maturing system. When you're in menopause, you've gone a year without a feminine period. It's not unexpected to encounter side effects like vaginal dryness and hot glimmers. Open up to your medical care supplier about the side effects you're encountering and what they mean for your personal satisfaction. They can prescribe medicines to deal with your side effects and make you more agreeable.

Chapter 2

VMS Menopause

VMS, or hot blazes and night sweats, are in many cases thought about the cardinal side effects of menopause. VMS are episodes of lavish intensity joined by perspiring and flushing, experienced transcendently around the head, neck, chest, and upper back. VMS is capable by most ladies during menopausal progress. In SWAN, 60-80% of ladies experience VMS eventually during the menopausal progress, with commonness rates changing by racial/ethnic group.1 Exploration from SWAN demonstrates that the event and recurrence of VMS top in the late perimenopause and early postmenopausal years,1 or quite a while encompassing the last feminine period. Notwithstanding, research from a scope of studies has shown that a sizable minority of ladies report VMS prior in midlife, before the beginning of period changes,2 and very much into their 60s and 70s, many years after the menopause transition.3, 4 Given the predominance and span of VMS among midlife ladies, it is basic to comprehend the hidden science of this side effect, the degree to which VMS might debilitate personal satisfaction, and whether VMS might act as a marker for other significant ailments.

Physiology of VMS

Conceptive chemicals

The physiology of hot blazes isn't completely perceived and logically addresses the interaction between various focal and fringe physiologic frameworks. Conceptive chemicals probably assume an essential part, as confirmed by the beginning of VMS happening with regards to the emotional regenerative chemical changes of the menopausal progress and by the restorative job of exogenous estrogen in their treatment. SWAN investigations show that degrees of endogenous chemicals are related to VMS. On a yearly premise, SWAN members (N=3,302) investigated their experience of VMS over the earlier two weeks and gave a blood test to estimation of estradiol (E2), follicle invigorating chemical (FSH), testosterone (T), dehydroepiandrosterone sulfate

(DHEAS), and sex chemical restricting globulin (SHBG). Thought about independently, higher FSH and lower E2 were related with a more prominent probability of revealing VMS (north of 5 years), while just higher FSH levels were related with VMS when the two chemicals were considered together.5

A subset of SWAN ladies (N=742) likewise partook in the SWAN Day to-day Chemical Review, which included yearly pee assortment over a total period (or a tantamount timeframe for ladies without feminine cycles) for evaluation of urinary FSH, luteinizing chemical (LH), the progesterone metabolite pregnanediol glucuronide (PdG), and estrone forms (E1C). Ladies likewise finished an everyday VMS journal during this time. In this examination, discoveries were like those in the full partner among ladies who had proof of hindered ovulatory action, with higher FSH and lower E1C related with a more prominent probability of revealing VMS.6 This example was not seen among ladies who had all the earmarks of being ovulatory, among whom the main chemical related to VMS was higher PdG levels. Taken together, these discoveries demonstrate that lower estrogen and higher FSH levels are related to VMS announcing, especially for ladies with anovulatory cycles. Be that as it may, while all perimenopausal ladies experience these hormonal changes, not all ladies have VMS. Consequently, other physiologic frameworks past the conceptive hub should be having an effect on everything.

Thermoregulatory

Driving models describe VMS, in some measure to a limited extent, as thermoregulatory heat scattering occasions. There is some proof of a restriction of the thermoneutral zone in suggestive postmenopausal ladies, or the zone wherein the center internal heat level is kept up without setting off thermoregulatory homeostatic systems like perspiring or shivering.7 Thusly, for indicative ladies, little variances in center internal heat level can surpass this zone and trigger intensity dissemination components like perspiring and fringe vasodilation (i.e., a hot blaze). Research showing that E2 organization decreases VMS and enlarges the thermoneutral zone adds backing to this model.8 While there is a piece of observational information to help this model, more examination is required. Different frameworks ensnared in the etiology of hot glimmers incorporate focal serotonergic, noradrenergic, narcotic, adrenal, and autonomic frameworks, as well as vascular cycles, however, little proof is accessible to obviously clarify their part in the beginning of hot flashes.9-13

Hereditary qualities

SWAN and different examinations have looked to portray the relationship between hereditary polymorphisms and VMS. Until this point, estrogen receptor (trauma center) polymorphisms and chosen single nucleotide polymorphisms (SNPs) of qualities engaged with the biosynthesis and digestion of various estrogens (i.e., E2, estrone, estriol) have been investigated. Variations in qualities that encode for trauma center alpha and in compounds engaged with union of and change among more and less strong estrogens have been found to anticipate the probability of VMS in the different racial/ethnic gatherings concentrated on in SWAN (n=1,538).14, 15 Despite the fact that there have been a few irregularities between discoveries, comparable outcomes have been seen in different examinations researching SNPs associated with combination and digestion of estrogens,16-19 as well as emergency room alpha.20 as a general rule, these affiliations persevere in the wake of adapting to other significant contributory elements, including conceptive chemical levels. Given the laid out changeability between race/ethnic gatherings in hereditary polymorphisms, SWAN results give a significant commitment to how we might interpret quality/VMS affiliations due to the consideration of enormous quantities of ladies from various racial/ethnic minority gatherings. Taken together, these outcomes recommend that the connection between VMS and hereditary polymorphisms might be because of polymorphisms that adjust sex steroid chemical movement. Nonetheless, it isn't known whether these hereditary determinants apply their belongings halfway in the cerebrum or incidentally on the autonomic sensory system, vasculature, or different frameworks possibly engaged with the beginning of VMS.

Risk factors for VMS

Race/Identity

VMS shows articulated racial/ethnic varieties. Of the five racial/ethnic gatherings concentrated on in SWAN, African American ladies were probably going to report VMS. All ladies were additionally bound to portray their VMS as vexatious, even in the wake of controlling for the expanded pace of revealing VMS among African American ladies. Caucasian and Hispanic ladies in SWAN are extensively comparable in their paces of detailing VMS. Notwithstanding, articulated variety across various ethnic gatherings of Hispanic ladies has been noted in SWAN, with the most noteworthy paces of VMS announced among Focal American ladies and the most reduced rates among Cuban women.[21] Chinese and Japanese ladies in SWAN are to the least extent liable to report VMS, with Japanese ladies to the least extent liable to report VMS and to portray them as bothersome.[1, 22]

The purposes behind these racial/ethnic contrasts are reasonable differed and not completely perceived. Albeit key elements related to VMS show articulated racial/ethnic variety, including BMI, E2 levels, smoking, chemical use, and financial position, racial/ethnic contrasts in VMS in SWAN continue subsequent to controlling for these factors.1 Others have proposed that the low degree of VMS among Asian versus Caucasian ladies is because of Asian ladies' generally high soy admission. Nonetheless, in SWAN, this doesn't give off an impression of being the case,1, 23 reliable with discoveries from randomized controlled preliminaries that have created blended or uncertain outcomes in regards to the utilization of soy or isoflavones for the administration of VMS.24-26 Besides, encountering and detailing any actual side effect, including VMS, is perplexing and impacted by a scope of perceptual and revealing cycles. Social varieties in how ladies experience, decipher, mark, and report VMS to others may likewise assume a part in noticed racial/ethnic contrasts in VMS.27

Weight

A key gamble factor for VMS is weight. For a long time, heftiness was believed to be defensive against VMS on the grounds that androgens are aromatized into estrogens in body fat.28 Ladies with more fat tissue would be supposed to have a lower chance of VMS in view of more elevated levels of estrogen. One critical finding from SWAN and other enormous observational examinations is that weight may be a gamble factor, as opposed to a defensive trademark, for VMS during the perimenopause and early postmenopause. For instance, in SWAN (N=3,302), ladies with no or rare VMS had a typical BMI of 28 kg/m2, while those with more successive VMS (having VMS no less than 6 days in the beyond two weeks) had a typical BMI of 31 kg/m2.1 This relationship among VMS and higher BMI persevered subsequent to controlling for related risk factors. Disclosures of a positive connection among BMI and VMS are all the more consistent with a thermoregulatory model of VMS, in which fat tissue goes about as a protector, forestalling the intensity dispersing activity of VMS, consequently expanding their event or seriousness. In any case, the systems liable for joins among corpulence and VMS are not perceived and may incorporate other physiologic components, including a potential job of other endocrine elements of fat tissue.29 Besides, the positive relationship between stoutness and VMS might be generally material to ladies prior to the menopausal change (e.g., in perimenopause or early postmenopause).30-34

The insightful methodologies used to analyze the relationship between corpulence and VMS basically utilize determined BMI, which envelops both lean and fat mass, and in this manner can't perceive the overall commitments of fat and lean mass as indicators of VMS. Since the commitment of fat tissue to take a chance for VMS might result from its thermoregulatory properties or its endocrine items, seeing explicitly the way that adiposity is connected with VMS is significant. SWAN investigations have analyzed the relationship of adiposity to VMS utilizing three unique methodologies. The first of these examinations analyzed adiposity as estimated by bioelectrical impedance investigation (BIA) (N=1,776), which yields proportions of both fat and lean mass. A higher all-out level of muscle versus fat, however not fit mass, was connected with an improved probability of VMS subsequent to controlling for frustrating elements like regenerative chemicals, smoking, race/identity, schooling, and negative affect.35 Every second investigation from SWAN used figured tomography (CT) proportions of stomach adiposity (N=461). CT yields proportions of complete stomach adiposity, including subcutaneous adiposity, or the fat tissue between the skin and the muscular strength wall, and instinctive adiposity, or the fat tissue behind the abs wall and in the peritoneal space around the organs. Outstandingly, subcutaneous fat is especially insulating.36 Results showed that higher stomach adiposity, and especially subcutaneous adiposity, was related to an improved probability of hot flashes.37 These affiliations were not represented by puzzling variables or conceptive chemicals (E2 and FSH). At last, a third investigation from SWAN used proportions of BIA north of four-year duration, consequently permitting assessment of progress in adiposity over the long haul corresponding to VMS (N=1,659). This examination is especially pertinent given that weight gain is normal during midlife.38 Discoveries showed that compared with ladies who kept up with stable muscle versus fat, gains in muscle versus fat over time were related to an improved probability of VMS at the resulting visit.39 These affiliations were free of perplexing elements and changes in conceptive chemicals. Taken together, these discoveries show that among perimenopausal and early postmenopausal ladies, adiposity was related to an improved probability of VMS, a seeing as steady with both a thermoregulatory model of VMS and furthermore an endocrine model of adiposity and VMS.

Wellbeing ways of behaving

The possible job of well-being ways of behaving in VMS has been exceptionally compelling. One of the most reliably noticed well-being ways of behaving related to VMS is smoking. In SWAN, throughout six years of follow-up, current smokers had a more than 60% improved probability of detailing VMS compared with nonsmokers,1 adapted to perplexing variables like training, BMI, menopausal status, and race/identity. As a matter of fact, SWAN results show that both dynamic smoking and detached smoke openness are related to a more prominent probability of VMS.23 It has been estimated that the relationship between smoking and VMS is because of the counter-estrogenic impacts of cigarette smoking.40 Nonetheless, testing this clarification is proof from SWAN demonstrating that distinctions in endogenous E2 levels didn't represent the relationship between smoking and VMS.23

Other eminent well-being ways of behaving, like dietary variables and actual work, have shown a lot more vulnerable relationship with VMS. In SWAN, dietary factors like all out kilocalorie, fat, fiber, caffeine, liquor admission, or explicit nutrient admission have not been related to VMS, subsequent to representing jumbling elements like training, smoking, and BMI.1, 23 Albeit beginning reports showed a gainful impact of the isoflavone, genistein, comparable to VMS,23 this affiliation was not seen in later longitudinal analyses.1 One more well-being conduct specifically compelling is physical activity.41 Active work has likewise not been in every case related to VMS in SWAN and different examinations, after change for bewildering factors.1, 41 It is striking that actual work might play double parts corresponding to VMS, emphatically affecting variables, for example, mindset and body weight, which might further develop VMS, yet additionally intensely raise center internal heat level, which could hypothetically build the event of VMS. Together, these SWAN examinations propose that smoking is the well-being conduct most plainly connected with VMS, with diet and actual work showing a lot more vulnerable or conflicting relationship with VMS.

Negative effect

Negative temperament (influence) has reliably been related to VMS across examinations. In SWAN (N=3302), more significant levels of tension, burdensome side effects, and saw pressure to concentrate on a section have been related to an improved probability of VMS happening over the resulting six years.1 As a matter of fact, the mental component generally reliably connected with hot glimmers is uneasiness, an affiliation that has been seen in SWAN and other studies.42 Notwithstanding an expansion in the event and recurrence of VMS, ladies with more noteworthy negative influence will more often than not rate their VMS as more troublesome, even subsequent to representing the higher recurrence of their VMS. The connections between bad effects and VMS are not completely perceived and may include a complicated interchange among physiologic and mental elements. It is deep-rooted that negative influence can impact side effect revealing, with a propensity towards raised side effect detailing with regards to negative affect.43 For instance, ladies with a more noteworthy aversion to actual side effects overall might be bound to hence report VMS.1 Exploration with physiological hot blaze screens has affirmed the significance of negative effects in the detailing of hot glimmers, showing a more noteworthy probability that hot blazes are accounted for when they are not recognized physiologically.44, 45 Nonetheless, the connection between bad effect and VMS is bidirectional, as VMS likewise impact mindset, as examined underneath.

Other social and segment factors

Various other social and mental elements have been related to an improved probability of VMS. Kid misuse and disregard are common in the SWAN populace and are related to a scope of poor physical and emotional wellness results. VMS is no exemption. Ladies who embraced a past filled with kid misuse or disregard (38% of the example evaluated) were bound to report VMS during the menopausal progress even subsequent to controlling for numerous variables, including negative effects, sociodemographic elements, and well-being behaviors.46 Another significant sociodemographic risk factor for VMS is low financial position. Ladies who are in lower financial positions, incorporating ladies with lower instructive achievement, lower pay, or who underwrite trouble paying for essentials are bound to report VMS comparative with their higher financial position counterparts.1 The explanations behind the relationship between financial position and VMS, an affiliation seen across studies, are not surely known. Lower financial position is related to smoking, higher BMI, higher saw pressure, and higher negative affect,47, 48, and is concentrated among specific minority racial/ethnic groups.49 Nonetheless, in SWAN, the relationship between low financial position and VMS couldn't be represented by any of these possibly puzzling elements. It is outstanding that the impact of low financial position or early openings, for example, youngster maltreatment on well-being is logically the consequence of various social, mental, and physiologic cycles working over a daily existence course, giving a test to making sense of these affiliations any arrangement of evaluations regulated at midlife.47, 50

Related personal satisfaction side effects

SWAN has examined the relationship between VMS and key personal satisfaction results that might be affected by the presence of VMS. These incorporate rest, state of mind, and mental capability. As every one of these side effect areas is canvassed independently in different segments of this exceptional release, we will momentarily examine accessible SWAN information that addresses explicitly the relationship between VMS and these normal side effects influencing personal satisfaction. In SWAN examinations, VMS has been unequivocally connected with decreased well-being related personal satisfaction (HRQL), despite the fact that the menopause stage itself was not related to HRQL.51, 52 The pessimistic relationship among VMS and HRQL is most grounded in those with more continuous VMS.51

Rest

SWAN results have major areas of strength for shown among VMS and saw rest aggravation in cross-sectional analyses,53 longitudinal examinations that follow ladies every year across the menopausal transition,54 and in day to day journal concentrates on that catch a more nitty gritty example of the nearby relationship between detailed VMS and rest problems.55 VMS have been related with all parts of seen rest unsettling influence that add to unfortunate rest coherence and quality, including nodding off, staying unconscious, and early-morning awakening.54 In all investigations, VMS revealing stands apart as a steady component that adds to detailing unfortunate rest subsequent to controlling for other significant prescient variables. This information is reliable with various different investigations that have comparably depicted areas of strength for a between revealed VMS and saw rest unsettling influence. The SWAN Rest Study has gathered broad information which will address the relationship between VMS and equitably estimated rest utilizing polysomnography (PSG). Consequences of continuous examinations bearing on the relationship among VMS and PSG-estimated rest are enthusiastically anticipated given the more dubious surviving writing on the relationship among VMS and dispassionately estimated rest boundaries.

State of mind

VMS and state of mind have all the earmarks of being connected in various and possibly complex ways. Beginning proof for joins among VMS and gloom comes from concentrates, for example, SWAN showing that elevated degrees of burdensome symptoms[56-58], as well as clinically critical depression[59-61], are generally normal during the perimenopause and early postmenopause when VMS is generally predominant. SWAN and different investigations have likewise found that perimenopausal ladies with VMS are bound to foster gloom following the beginning of VMS than are perimenopausal ladies without VMS,[56, 59-64] albeit these connections might be because of different variables related to having a burdensome episode, for example, an earlier history of nervousness problem and unpleasant life events.[59]

Studies have demonstrated the way that VMS can both go before and follow, as well as happen simultaneously with, depression,65 showing that the connection between VMS and misery might be made sense of by various different causal pathways. At the point when gloom co-happens with or follows VMS, VMS might bring about temperament aggravation on the grounds that VMS can disable rest, which is a significant gamble factor for melancholy. On the other hand, VMS might be an underlying suggestive appearance of bothers in brain frameworks that likewise underlie despondency. Circuitous proof proposes that the serotonergic and noradrenergic frameworks, synapse frameworks usually connected to despondency, might be engaged with the etiology of VMS,10-13, 66 raising the likelihood that focal sensory system processes add to both VMS and

sadness weakness.

In any case, numerous ladies with VMS don't encounter wretchedness. The perception that VMS happens without a trace of wretchedness and that downturn happens in midlife ladies without VMS shows that neither one of the circumstances is expected for the other side effect to

show. Further examination is justified to comprehend the causal connection between these two normal midlife side effects.

Mental capability

SWAN examinations (n=2362) have shown that there is a transient decrement in mental execution during perimenopause, which is described by a decreased capacity to discover that thusly settle as ladies become postmenopausal.67 Extra SWAN examinations (n=1903) have demonstrated that this transient decrement isn't made sense of by VMS.68 This information is steady with some,69 however not all,70 other more modest investigations which comparably found a shortfall of a relationship among VMS and verbal memory execution when VMS are estimated by self-report. Interestingly, concentrating on estimating VMS unbiasedly show a converse connection among's VMS and mental performance,71 proposing that physiologic changes in basic VMS might be connected straightforwardly and halfway to mental capability.

Go to:

Arising joins among VMS and sickness results

VMS has customarily been conceptualized as a significant personal satisfaction issue during the menopausal change, and they have commonly not been expected to have explicit ramifications for actual well-being. In any case, arising research from SWAN and different examinations has started to raise doubt about this suspicion.

Cardiovascular gamble

Introductory work from a few enormous preliminaries of chemical treatment, including the Ladies' Wellbeing Drive (WHI) and the Heart and Estrogen Substitution Study (HERS), proposed joins among VMS and cardiovascular infection (CVD) risk. In the two examinations, the raised coronary illness occasion risk related to chemical treatment use was most noteworthy among ladies announcing moderate to extreme VMS at the review passage, and in WHI, the more established ladies with VMS.72, 73 We have followed up on these underlying perceptions in SWAN, investigating expected joins among VMS and CVD. A lot of this examination has been led with regards to the SWAN Heart Study (N=588), a subordinate review to SWAN which gathered information on a few proportions of subclinical CVD, including brachial corridor stream interceded widening, a marker of endothelial brokenness; coronary course and aortic calcification, proportions of calcified plaques in these blood vessel beds; and carotid intima-media thickness (IMT), a deeply grounded marker of atherosclerosis. These subclinical CVD measures are helpful to comprehend the risk for CVD among illness-free people, as each of the three measures has been tentatively connected with raised cardiovascular occasion rates among people without clinical CVD.74-76 Discoveries showed that ladies detailing hot glimmers and account of IMT, more regular hot blazes, had less fortunate endothelial capability, more noteworthy aortic calcification, and more noteworthy IMT when contrasted with their partners without hot flashes.77, 78 These affiliations persevered in the wake of controlling for perplexing segments and other referred to cardiovascular gamble factors as well as E2 levels. Discoveries for night sweats were like those for hot glimmers, yet at the same fairly lessened. Eminently, the relationship between hot glimmers and IMT was generally articulated for ladies who were overweight or fat as well concerning ladies who experienced hot moves quickly over different yearly visits, recommending that hot blazes might be generally educational as for CVD risk when they are diligent and when they happen in people with other CVD risk factors, like stoutness. The exact explanations behind and nature of the relationship between VMS and CVD risk require further examination and elucidation. In any case, one understanding of these discoveries is that hot glimmers might be a suggestive sign of fundamental unfavorable changes in a lady's vasculature.

Bone wellbeing

Arising research from SWAN and different investigations has connected VMS and bone mineral thickness and bone turnover. In the first of these SWAN examinations (N=2213), ladies detailing VMS had lower bone mineral

density.79 This affiliation was seen across ladies of all menopausal stages in the example, especially among the postmenopausal ladies. The relationship between VMS and bone mineral thickness changed by unambiguous bone site studies, generally evident at the lumbar spine and hip among postmenopausal ladies, and at the femoral neck among ladies prior to the menopausal progress. In a moment set of SWAN examinations (N=2283), the event of VMS was additionally analyzed comparable to an exceptionally delicate marker of bone turnover, urinary N-telopeptide. In these examinations, perimenopausal and postmenopausal ladies with VMS had higher bone turnover (higher urinary N-telopeptide) than their partners without VMS.80 In the two examinations of bone thickness and bone turnover, affiliations generally endured subsequent to controlling for likely confounders, in spite of the fact that E2 and FSH levels represented some, yet not these affiliations. The expected purposes behind the relationship between VMS and bone well-being require further examination, including an investigation of the possible commitment of the hypothalamic-pituitary-adrenal hub and the thoughtful apprehensive system.79 Nonetheless, these outcomes recommend that VMS might be a significant mark of some part of declining ovarian capability that isn't caught by feminine cycle changes or yearly conceptive chemical levels.

Rundown and Ends

SWAN has yielded special experiences about VMS, the cardinal side effect of menopause. We have discovered that VMS is capable by most midlife ladies, yet show articulated racial/ethnic contrasts that can't be made sense of by other realized VMS risk factors. Key gamble factors for VMS incorporate low schooling, smoking, and negative effect. Weight, recently remembered to be defensive against VMS, is really a gamble factor for VMS among perimenopausal and early postmenopausal ladies. Further, VMS is related to more unfortunate personal satisfaction, pessimistic temperament, and rest issues during midlife. The relationship between VMS and temperament is mind-boggling, bidirectional, and potentially made sense of by various pathways, including rest and brain components. At last, arising data from SWAN demonstrates that VMS might be connected to specific unfriendly actual well-being results, including subclinical cardiovascular infection and lower bone thickness. In this way, SWAN has been a rich wellspring of data about its normal and frequently irksome midlife side effects. Continuous discoveries from SWAN will keep on yielding significant data about VMS in the years to come.

Chapter 3

Paresthesia

What is paresthesia?

"Paresthesia" is the specialized term for the impression of shivering, consuming, pricking or prickling, skin-slithering, tingling, "tingling sensation" or deadness on or just under your skin. It can influence puts on and all through your body and occurs without an external reason or caution.

Paresthesia (some of the time known as "paresthesia of skin") is an extremely normal encounter. Everybody encounters it sooner or later, and it can occur for some reasons. A significant number of the normal causes are innocuous and are only an impression of how your body functions regularly. However, at times, paresthesia can flag a clinical issue.

There are two principal types of paresthesia:

- **Transient (transitory):** This is the more normal sort. As the name proposes, it doesn't keep going long. A model would be a concise shivering or a tingling sensation feeling in your leg on the off chance that you sat a specific excessively lengthy. When you broaden your leg, the inclination ought to get back to business as usual.
- **Relentless (constant):** This is when paresthesia waits and doesn't disappear. By and large a side effect of issues might require clinical consideration. Conditions like carpal passage disorder or cubital passage disorder are generally minor ways that persevering paresthesia can occur. However, you can likewise have steady paresthesia from an absence of flow or nerve harm, the two of which are in many cases more serious.

What is paresthesia?

"Paresthesia" is the specialized term for the impression of shivering, consuming, pricking or prickling, skin-slithering, tingling, "tingling sensation" or deadness on or just under your skin. It can influence puts on and all through your body and occurs without an external reason or caution.

Paresthesia (in some cases known as "paresthesia of skin") is an exceptionally normal encounter. Everybody encounters it sooner or later, and it can occur for some reasons. A large number of the normal causes are innocuous and are only an impression of how your body functions regularly. Be that as it may, at times, paresthesia can flag a clinical issue.

There are two fundamental types of paresthesia:

- **Transient (brief):** This is the more normal sort. As the name proposes, it doesn't keep going long. A model would be a short shivering or a tingling sensation feeling in your leg in the event that you sat for a specific excessively lengthy. When you broaden your leg, the inclination ought to get back to business as usual.
- **Constant (ongoing):** This is when paresthesia waits and doesn't disappear. For the most part, a side effect of issues might require clinical consideration.

Conditions like carpal passage disorder or cubital passage disorder are moderately minor ways that steady paresthesia can occur. However, you can likewise have persevering paresthesia from an absence of dissemination or nerve harm, the two of which are much of the time more serious.

What are the most well-known reasons for paresthesia?

Transient and determined paresthesias will more often than not have altogether different causes.

Transient paresthesia

Transient paresthesia is exceptionally normal, and it's generally innocuous. It regularly happens in view of body situating that comes down on a nerve or cutoff points bloodstream (like collapsing a wrinkle into a hose to hold fluid back from coursing through). That can cause the impacted body part to "nod off" (the specialized term for this is "obdormition"). Paresthesia is the sensation of a tingling sensation that happens when you change position and delivery the strain on the nerve or veins in that body part.

Transient paresthesia can likewise occur assuming you hit specific body parts against strong articles. For instance, knocking something with your elbow can cause a sharp, shock-like sensation of shivering or torment in your ulnar nerve. That is known as "hitting your amusing bone," as your ulnar nerve is at the lower end of your really upper arm bone, your humerus.

A few different reasons for transient paresthesia include:

- Lack of hydration.
- Formication (a touch-based mind flight that feels like bugs slithering on your skin).
- Hyperventilation.
- Headaches.
- Nerve pressure disorders, like carpal passage condition and cubital passage disorder (these can become determined when they're moderate or extreme).
- Fits of anxiety.
- Renaud's disorder.

- Seizures.
- Whiplash.
- Tireless paresthesia

Tireless paresthesia implies it's steady or happens regularly. It's bound to be from serious purposes, which will more often than not fall into specific classes.

Circulatory causes

One general classification is circulatory causes. An absence of dissemination that influences your nerves can disturb how those nerves convey signs to and from your mind. That can cause paresthesia.

Thoracic outlet disorder is an illustration of a circulatory condition that might cause paresthesia. At the point when it's constant, Reynaud's condition can likewise be a type of circulatory-related paresthesia.

Sensory system causes

Neurological causes can include your mind, spinal rope, or nerves anyplace in your body. A few instances of neurological causes include:

- Ataxia-telangiectasia.
- Mind growths.
- Mind drains.
- Charcot-Marie-Tooth infection.
- Head wounds, like blackouts and horrendous cerebrum wounds (TBIs).
- Herniated plates.
- Nerve harm from consumption or frostbite.
- Neuralgia (nerve torment) sicknesses, including occipital neuralgia and trigeminal neuralgia.
- Fringe neuropathy.
- Squeezed nerves or radiculopathy.
- Spinal stenosis.
- Strokes or transient ischemic assaults (TIAs).

Metabolic and endocrine causes

Metabolic and endocrine causes incorporate a lack of nutrients, conditions that influence specific chemicals from there, the sky is the limit. Models include:

- Diabetes-related neuropathy (nerve harm).
- Electrolyte lopsided characteristics.
- Low glucose (hypoglycemia).
- Low parathyroid capability (hypoparathyroidism).
- Low thyroid capability (hypothyroidism).
- Menopause.
- Vitamin B1 (thiamine) inadequacy (otherwise called beriberi), B5 lack, B6 inadequacy,d B12 lack.

Irresistible illnesses

Irresistible illnesses can normally cause paresthesia when they influence nerves or portions of your mind. Instances of these circumstances include:

- Any disease that can influence your cerebrum and cause encephalitis or meningitis.
- Guillain-Barré disorder.

- Hansen's illness (sickness).
- Herpes simplex infection.
- Herpes zoster infection (shingles).
- Human immunodeficiency infection (HIV).
- Lyme sickness.
- Syphilis.

Immune system and provocative sicknesses

Immune system conditions are the point at which your invulnerable framework assaults portions of your own body. Paresthesia is one of the potential side effects of an immune system condition that goes after your nerves. Provocative circumstances can likewise cause expanding and tissue changes that influence nerves. These circumstances can include:

- Fibromyalgia.
- Lupus.
- Numerous sclerosis.
- Rheumatoid joint inflammation.
- Sjögren's disorder.
- Cross-over myelitis.

Harmful impacts

In the same way as other tissues in your body, your sensory system is defenseless against poisons and toxic substances. Instances of harmful wellsprings of paresthesia include:

- Arsenic harming.
- Carbon monoxide harming.
- Chemotherapy.
- Lead harming.
- Mercury harming.
- Neuropathy from liquor use jumble.
- Radiation affliction or consumption.
- Snake nibbles.
- Bug nibbles.
- Scorpion stings.
- Venomous stings/nibbles from different creatures.

Different causes

Different circumstances can likewise cause paresthesia. These can include organ issues or conditions that don't fall under the ones referenced previously. A couple of models include:

- Amyloidosis.
- Porphyria.
- Uremia.

Care And Treatment

How is paresthesia treated?

A few types of paresthesia particularly transient structures like an appendage nodding off don't require treatment. However, numerous different types of paresthesia might require treatment. The medicines rely upon basic reason, and that implies the medicines can change generally. Your medical care supplier is the best individual to educate you regarding the potential therapies which they suggest.

What are the potential confusions or dangers of not treating it?

Most reasons for paresthesia need treatment. A large number of these circumstances, particularly course-related related and neurological causes, are perilous or dangerous without treatment. Different circumstances that cause it, while not perilous, are troublesome and can adversely influence your personal satisfaction without treatment.

You ought to converse with a medical services supplier assuming you have paresthesia that influences a similar body part on the two sides, like your hands or feet. You ought to likewise converse with a supplier on the off chance that you regularly have paresthesia that isn't pose/body position-related. They see what's causing your paresthesia and whether it needs treatment.

What's the contrast between paresthesia and deadness?

Deadness is the point at which you can't feel sensations in the impacted region. Paresthesia is a sensation you might feel when there's a disturbance in your feeling of touch in the impacted region.

Paresthesia and deadness arc likc ncighbors with regard to actual sensations. You frequently feel paresthesia not long before deadness sets in, or paresthesia can be what you feel when sensation returns.

Note

Paresthesia is something that everybody encounters sooner or later in their life. More often than not, it's from straightforward, innocuous reasons like sitting in a place that makes your leg nod off or dozing on your hand for a lengthy period, causing it to feel numb for some time.

However, paresthesia can likewise flag more serious ailments. Assuming you have paresthesia that continues to occur for obscure reasons, or then again in the event that it occurs with different side effects, you ought to converse with your essential consideration supplier or another medical services supplier. They can nail down what's causing your paresthesia and assist you with understanding the reason why it's working out and what regardless should be finished about it.

Chapter 4

Premenstrual syndrome (PMS)

What is premenstrual disorder (PMS)?

Premenstrual condition, or PMS, depicts side effects that appear before your period. Side effects can be founded on feelings like touchiness or discouragement, or you might have actual side effects like bosom torment or bulging. These side effects normally emerge one to about fourteen days before you start your period and return simultaneously every month.

What is the distinction between PMS and PMDD?

Premenstrual dysphoric problem (PMDD) is a serious and possibly incapacitating type of PMS. Around 2% of individuals who discharge have PMDD. With PMDD, you experience PMS side effects yet with substantially more power, particularly with regard to profound reactions and your mindset. You're bound to encounter outrage, serious sorrow, and tension with PMDD than with PMS.

How normal is PMS?

In spite of the fact that it's not unexpected to have one or a couple of premenstrual side effects, clinically huge PMS happens in simply 3% to 8% percent of individuals who bleed.

Side effects And Causes

What are the signs and side effects of premenstrual disorder?

It's normal with PMS to encounter different side effects that adversely influence your body and your profound prosperity. The side effects related to PMS aren't unsurprising all of the time. The side effects you notice in your 20s might be not the same as the ones you experience in your 30s and 40s.

What is unsurprising is the timing. A throbbing painfulness or sensations of touchiness that routinely go before your period and afterward get better a while later are an indication of PMS.

Actual side effects

The most well-known actual indications of PMS are a sensation of totality in your stomach (swelling) and weariness. Different side effects include:

- Cramps.
- Skin break-out eruptions.
- Bosom delicacy.
- Migraines.

Profound side effects

Sensations of peevishness and emotional episodes are the most widely recognized profound marks of PMS. Different side effects include:

- Changes in your sex drive.
- Feeling restless, miserable, or discouraged.
- Cerebrum mist, or experiencing difficulty concentrating.

- Food desires or expanded/diminished craving.
- Laying down for continuous rests or experiencing difficulty dozing (sleep deprivation).
- Decreased interest in exercises.

The profound cost that PMS takes can make you pull out from loved ones. It can heighten gloomy sentiments, making it simpler to suddenly erupt toward others.

What is the connection between PMS and premenstrual worsening (PME)?

PMS imparts side effects to numerous different circumstances. These common side effects frequently deteriorate (compound) before your period. These circumstances include:

- **Wretchedness and nervousness:** Emotional episodes, sensations of bitterness, peevishness, and confinement might get more extraordinary around your period.
- **Myalgic encephalomyelitis/constant weariness disorder (ME/CFS):** Exhaustion and joint and muscle agony might strengthen in long stretches of

- time paving the way to your period. With ME/CFS, you're additionally bound to early experience weighty feminine draining and go through menopause.
- **Bad-tempered inside disorder (IBS):** Side effects like bulging, gas, and issues can deteriorate close to PMS.

Significant during determination to preclude conditions share side effects with PMS. Your medical services supplier will assist you with distinguishing whether your side effects are indications of PMS just or on the other hand in the event that you have a condition that feels more regrettable in light of the fact that you're going to discharge.

What causes premenstrual disorder?

The reasons for PMS are obscure. It's conceivable that chemical changes connected with your period make certain individuals experience PMS side effects. Side effects ordinarily appear after ovulation, when your ovaries discharge an egg. Your levels of the chemicals estrogen and progesterone plunge close to this time. Side effects frequently disappear a couple of days after your period, when your chemical levels begin to rise once more. These chemical vacillations might be to be faulted for PMS.

Determination And Tests

How is premenstrual disorder analyzed?

Your medical care supplier will get some information about what side effects you have when you have them and what they mean for your life. It's generally expected to encounter a terrible side effect or two every so often before your period, however, this isn't equivalent to PMS.

For a PMS determination, your supplier will affirm that you have no less than one side effect related to PMS that happens in something like five days of your feminine cycle and afterward disappears in no less than four days after your period closes. These side effects should repeat for somewhere around three monthly cycles for an authority finding.

Questions your supplier might ask include:

How long pass between one period and another?

How long do you drain?

How long are light, medium, or weighty?

What side effects do you have?

When do your side effects appear/disappear?

When are your side effects milder/more serious?

Could you at any point tell me when your side effects are going to begin? In what way?

Do your side effects impede your life? In what way?

Your supplier may likewise get some information about your clinical history and the drugs you're taking to preclude factors other than PMS that might be causing your side effects. They might get some information about your family's clinical history, as well, since many circumstances (like state of mind issues) run in families. Your supplier will preclude causes like:

- Tension.
- Sadness.
- Perimenopause (the temporary time frame before menopause).
- Constant weakness condition.
- Thyroid problems (ex. hyperthyroidism).

- Prescriptions you're taking.

The Executives And Treatments

Is there a solution for premenstrual conditions?

No. In any case, your side effects will ultimately disappear once you experience menopause and never again have periods. Up to that point, there's a bounty you can do to deal with your side effects so they don't disturb your life. Monitor when you will generally see side effects, and observe the medicines that alleviate them. Put them to utilize every month when your side effects generally start.

How might I oversee side effects?

You can as a rule oversee gentle side effects with way-of-life changes and over-the-counter (OTC) drugs. More serious side effects might require a remedy from your supplier.

Prescriptions

NSAIDs: Nonsteroidal mitigating drugs (NSAIDs) can ease bosom torment and feminine issues assuming you take them during your period or around when your side effects start. Choices incorporate Ibuprofen (Advil®, Motrin IB®), Naproxen sodium (Aleve®), Acetaminophen (Tylenol®), and Headache medicine. You can buy them over the counter, or your supplier can recommend a more grounded measurement in the event that your side effects are extreme.

- **Hormonal contraception:** Prescriptions that keep you from ovulating can assuage unsavory actual side effects, similar to delicacy and agony. It might take a trial and error at first to sort out what sort of contraception helps you most. Choices incorporate conception prevention pills, the fix, and the ring (NuvaRing®).

- **Antidepressants and against tension meds:** Specific serotonin reuptake inhibitors (SSRIs) are the most widely recognized kinds of upper endorsed to treat the state of mind-related issues related to PMS. Choices incorporate fluoxetine (Prozac®, Sarafem®), paroxetine (Paxil®, Pexeva®) and sertraline (Zoloft®). Take them just as coordinated by your supplier.

- **Diuretics:** Diuretics can alleviate side effects like swelling and bosom delicacy.
- **Way of life changes:** You can adjust your way of life to ease agony and battle the state of mind-related side effects of PMS.
- **Normal activity:** Moderate cardiworkoutut (running, lively strolling, cycling, or swimming) for 30 minutes daily can alleviate pressure and lift youmindsetet. The advantages lasted past 30 minutes.
- **Solid eating routine:** Eating a greater amount of certain food varieties and less of others can battle PMS side effects. Eat less pungent, greasy, and sweet food varieties, and drink less jazzed and cocktails fourteen days before your period. During your period, eat six little dinners daily rather than three major ones. Or on the other hand, eat three little feasts and three little tidbits. Smart dieting is really great for your state of mind and your stomach. Scattering your feasts forestalls inside inconveniences, similar to obstruction.

- **A lot of rest:** Getting something like eight hours of rest can decrease sensations of touchiness. Awakening and heading to sleep simultaneously every day adds the additional advantage of adjusting your inner clock so that you're less inclined to feel grumpy over the course of the day.
- **Unwinding works out:** Yoga, contemplation and breathing activities ease pressure and battle the touchiness and bitterness that frequently go with PMS.
-

Nutrients, minerals, and enhancements

Nutrients, minerals, and natural enhancements aren't controlled by the FDA how over-the-counter and physician-endorsed drugs are, so it's really smart to check with a medical services supplier prior to taking them. In any case, there's some proof that they can assist with PMS.

- **Calcium:** Exploration recommends that calcium can further develop side effects like weariness, food desires, and even misery. You can get calcium from dairy items (milk, eggs, yogurt), food sources with calcium added (a few oats and bread), and enhancements.

- **Magnesium:** There's contending proof about whether magnesium assists with PMS side effects, similar to migraines, stress, and tension. You can get magnesium from mixed greens, nuts, entire grains, and enhancements.

- **Vitamin B6:** A few examinations have demonstrated the way that Vitamin B6 can further develop side effects connected with gentle and direct PMS. You can get Vitamin B6 from fish, poultry, potatoes, and non-citrus leafy foods.

- **Omega-3 and Omega-6:** A few investigations have shown that Omega-3 and Omega - 6 unsaturated fats can ease PMS side effects. You can get Omega-3 and Omega-6 from fish, flaxseed, nuts, salad greens, and enhancements.

- **Natural enhancements:** A few homegrown cures are utilized to free the side effects from PMS, with changing levels of proof. These incorporate dark cohosh, dried chaste berry, and evening primrose oil. Converse with your supplier prior to beginning

-

homegrown enhancements to guarantee it's protected and that you're taking the perfect sum.

Anticipation

How might I forestall premenstrual disorder?

You can't forestall PMS, however, you can oversee side effects with the way of life changes, drugs, or a mix of both.

Viewpoint/Guess

What might I at any point expect assuming I have premenstrual disorder?

PMS is normal enough that many individuals acknowledge it as a burden during "that time" that they need to live with. Yet, you don't need to persevere through side effects that disturb your life. Frequently, you can deal with your side effects with drugs and way of life changes. Assuming nothing you're doing is having a sufficiently large effect, see your supplier seek medicines that can help.

Living With

When would it be a good idea for me to see my medical care supplier?

See your supplier on the off chance that you can't get alleviation from your PMS side effects. To benefit from your visit, come to your arrangement arranged to talk about your side effects and your period exhaustively. Track your period and side effect history on a schedule, organizer, or application. Be ready to share data about your period start and stop dates and your side effects (counting how gentle or serious) for somewhere around two sequential periods.

What inquiries would it be advisable for me to pose to my supplier?

Are my side effects simply connected with PMS or might they at any point be an indication of something different?

What way of life changes could you prescribe to oversee side effects?

How might I advise whether I really want a solution to facilitate my side effects?

Could you prescribe natural enhancements to ease PMS side effects?

How could I proactively deal with my PMS side effects?

Oftentimes Got clarification on some things

How would you fix the premenstrual condition?

You can't fix PMS, yet you can oversee it with the way of life changes and prescriptions. A definitive PMS "fix" is menopause, when you never again get periods or the side effects that go with them.

How long does PMS endure before you get your period?

The beginning of PMS side effects fluctuates. For a PMS finding, you ought to see side effects in the span of five days prior to beginning your period. However, the timing isn't precise 100% of the time. You might begin to see side effects fourteen days before your period or two days before your period. Focus on your examples.

What is PME and how can it connect with my period?

PME is short for premenstrual worsening. Assuming you have conditions that share side effects with PMS, you might see that they deteriorate around your period. Converse with your supplier about how your side effects change in light of your period.

Note

Since premenstrual disorder is normal doesn't imply that you need to endure the unsavory side effects it causes. Focus on any throbbing painfulness or state of mind changes that occur around your period that might be indications of PMS. Assuming they're obstructing your prosperity, have a go at changing around your propensities and assuming control of non-prescription drugs that can ease side effects. In the event that that doesn't work, see a medical services supplier to seek the therapy you really want.

Chapter 5

Peri-Menopausal Symptoms

What is perimenopause?

Perimenopause (likewise alluded to as the menopause change) is the point at which your body begins progressing to menopause. During this progress, your ovaries start creating fewer chemicals, making your feminine cycle become sporadic or unpredictable. Right now, your body is advancing close to the furthest limit of your regenerative years.

Perimenopause might start as soon as your mid-30s or as late as your mid-50s. Certain individuals are in perimenopause for just a brief time frame. However, for the overwhelming majority, it endures four to eight years. The term perimenopause basically portrays when your cycles are as of now not unsurprising.

Other actual changes and side effects can happen as your body acclimates to various chemical levels. During perimenopause, your richness is declining, however, you all things considered can become pregnant. The side effects of perimenopause, the age it starts and how lengthy it endures will change between ladies. You're out of perimenopause and into menopause whenever you've had 12 continuous months without a feminine period.

What is the distinction between perimenopause and menopause?

Perimenopause is a momentary time that finishes in menopause. Menopause implies your periods have finished. At the point when you have no period for an entire year, you have formally arrived at menopause.

For what reason does perimenopause occur?

Your ovaries start to deliver less estrogen as you age in an arrangement to quit delivering eggs altogether. Eventually, your body is planning to change to menopause, when you lose the capacity to get pregnant.

It's a characteristic and ordinary movement in a lady's regenerative cycle.

What is the distinction between perimenopause and menopause?

Perimenopause is a temporary time that closes in menopause. Menopause implies your periods have finished. At the point when you have no feminine cycle for an entire year, you have formally arrived at menopause.

For what reason does perimenopause occur?

Your ovaries start to create less estrogen as you age in readiness to quit delivering eggs altogether. Eventually, your body is planning to change to menopause, when you lose the capacity to get pregnant. It's a characteristic and typical movement in a lady's conceptive cycle.

What are the hormonal changes during perimenopause?

The hormonal changes you experience during perimenopause are generally achieved by declining estrogen levels. Your ovaries make estrogen, which assumes an imperative part in keeping up with the regenerative framework. When you enter perimenopause, your estrogen levels begin to diminish. As estrogen diminishes, it loses the offset with progesterone, another chemical produces by the ovaries. These two chemicals together are liable for ovulation and monthly cycle. It's typical for compound levels to waver during perimenopause to go all over like a rollercoaster.

At the point when you arrive at menopause, your body makes so little estrogen that your ovaries never again discharge eggs. As of now, you quit having your period.

What are the primary indications of perimenopause?

By and large, the primary indication of perimenopause is unpredictable periods. The vast majority will go from having genuinely unsurprising periods to unusual cycles. Many individuals likewise experience the most well-known indications of menopause like hot blazes and vaginal dryness (vaginal decay) genuinely right on time into the menopause progress.

Side effects And Causes

What are the side effects of perimenopause?

Your body has been delivering estrogen since pubescence. When your estrogen levels start to decline, your body needs to conform to the progressions in chemicals.

The side effects shift, yet the vast majority experience somewhere around one of the accompanying:

- Unpredictable periods or skipping periods.
- Periods that are heavier or lighter than expected.
- Hot glimmers (an unexpected sensation of warmth that spreads across your body).
- Vaginal dryness and anxiety during sex.
- Urinary desperation (expecting to pee all the more habitually).

Rest issues (a sleeping disorder).

Changes in the state of mind like peevishness, melancholy or emotional episodes.

The time span you have side effects of perimenopause can change between a couple of months to numerous years. The lessening in estrogen additionally also prompt bone loss or changing cholesterol levels. Keep on having customary tests with your medical care supplier to watch out for your well-being.

How are periods during perimenopause?

Your body is creating fewer of the chemicals that assist you with ovulating, so your periods can become sporadic. Your feminine cycle could turn out to be longer or more limited than expected. Your drainageVaginal dryness and tension during sex.Vaginal dryness and tension during sex. could likewise be heavier or lighter than typical. Certain individuals likewise notice an adjustment inVaginal dryness and tension during sex. their premenstrual syndrome (PMS) side effects.

How can I tell whether changes in my periods are typical perimenopausal side effects or something to be worried about?

Sporadic periods are normal and typical during perimenopause, yet different circumstances can cause irregularities in female dying. In the event that any of the accompanying circumstances concern you, see a medical care provider to rule out different causes.

- Your periods are changing to turn out to be extremely weighty or joined by blood clusters.
- Your last period was a few days longer than expected.
- You spot or drain after your period.
- You experience spotting after sex.
- Your periods happen closer together.

Possible reasons for unusual draining includes: perimenopausal hormonal awkwardness, contamination, pregnancy-related dying, fibroids, blood-thickening issues, endometrial polyps, premature delivery, taking blood thinners, or disease.

Do you actually ovulate during perimenopause?

On the off chance that you're actually getting a period, even a sporadic one, you're actually ovulating. Until you haven't discharged for 12 consecutive months, you ought to expect that your body is as yet ovulating (delivering eggs).

Conclusion And Tests

How is perimenopause analyzed?

You don't necessarily, in every case, need to see a medical services supplier for a perimenopause finding. Many individuals notice and endure the progressions in their bodies without a conventional finding. On the off chance that you have side effects that impede your day-to-day activities, see a medical services supplier.

You ought to connect with your medical services supplier immediately on the off chance that you have:

- Blood clumps in the feminine release.
- Spotting between periods
- Vaginal drainage after sex

Profound side effects slow down your capacity to work consistently.

What FSH level means perimenopause?

FSH (follicle invigorating chemical) is a chemical delivered by the pituitary organ — the organ situated at the foundation of your mind. It invigorates the ovaries to deliver an egg during ovulation. Testing your FSH level can assist with affirming menopause has begun. A reliably elevated degree of FSH can show menopause. Notwithstanding, FSH tests can be deceiving in light of the fact that during perimenopause your chemicals rise and fall whimsically. Certain prescriptions, similar to conception prevention pills or chemical treatment, disrupt chemical levels and will influence the consequences of any chemical tests. Overactive thyroid and high prolactin can likewise change those outcomes.

The executives And Treatments

Will perimenopause be dealt with?

There isn't any treatment to stop perimenopause. Perimenopause is a trademark piece of life. The "fix" for perimenopause happens when your periods stop and you enter menopause.

However, your medical services supplier might suggest over-the-counter or remedy perimenopause therapy to assist with facilitating side effects. Your supplier might suggest:

- **Antidepressants:** These drugs assist with temperament swings or sorrow.

Conception prevention pills. These drugs settle your chemical levels and commonly alleviate side effects.

- **Estrogen treatment:** This treatment settles estrogen levels. You might accept estrogen treatment as a cream, gel, fix, or swallowable pill.
- **Gabapentin (Neurontin®):** This medication is a seizure drug that likewise eases hot blazes for certain ladies.

- **Vaginal creams:** Your supplier can educate you concerning solutions and over-the-counter choices. Treatment can diminish torment connected with sex and alleviate vaginal dryness.

Your medical care supplier will examine the dangers and advantages of perimenopause therapy with you and suggest the most ideal choice in light of your necessities. A certain way of life changes like eating a solid eating regimen, light activity, and keeping away from food sources or exercises that trigger hot glimmers can likewise help.

What is the chemical treatment?

Chemical treatment can assist with easing a few side effects of perimenopause. As a general rule, medical care suppliers prescribe that individuals who pick to utilize chemical treatment start it no less than 10 years starting menopause side effects, and use it for under five years. Estrogen and chemicals have been connected to an expanded gamble of heart issues and a few kinds of bosom malignant growth.

Talk with your medical services supplier to ensure you comprehend the dangers and advantages of chemical treatment as a therapy for perimenopause.

What are the dangers of chemical treatment?

Treating perimenopause with chemical treatment can build your gamble for the accompanying circumstances:

- Uterine malignant growth.
- Stroke.
- Coronary episode.
- Blood clusters.
- Gallbladder illness.

How might I deal with my perimenopause side effects at home?

You might decide to oversee perimenopause side effects at home. To alleviate side effects, you can:

- Eat an eating routine loaded with natural products, vegetables, entire grains, lean protein, and sound fats.
-

- Perform weight-bearing activities like strolling, climbing, or strength preparing.
- Further develop rest cleanliness by trying not to screens and do loosening up exercises before bed.

Limit liquor and caffeine.

- Practice contemplation or other pressure the executives procedures.
- Stop smoking.
- Get in shape whenever demonstrated. Weight reduction diminishes hot blazes and night sweats and further develops your energy level.

Avoidance

What can place you into perimenopause early?

Certain variables are connected to early perimenopause. These include:

- Smoking or utilizing tobacco items.
- A family background of early menopause.
- A past filled with disease treatment.

Assuming you've had your uterus or ovaries eliminated.

How might I lessen my gamble of perimenopause confusions?

Sporadic periods are the most widely recognized side effect of perimenopause. Yet, it's vital to know when to converse with your medical services supplier about your periods. In some cases, unpredictable draining can highlight a basic issue.

You can bring down your gamble of entanglements by looking for treatment when important. Converse with your medical care supplier if you:

- Drain for over seven days straight.
- Drain between periods.
- Change cushions or tampons each one to two hours.
- Have periods more as often as possible than at regular intervals.

Viewpoint/Visualization

Are there any wellbeing chances related with perimenopause?

There are wellbeing chances related with menopause, which happens just after perimenopause.

Estrogen assumes a significant part in saving your bones. Osteoporosis is a condition where the internal parts of your bones become not so much thick but rather more delicate. This expands your gamble for bone breaks. Your medical care supplier might suggest a multivitamin, calcium supplement, additional vitamin D, or more weight-bearing activities.

Individuals in menopause are likewise at an expanded gamble for coronary illness and other cardiovascular medical issue.

Might I at any point get pregnant on the off chance that I am in perimenopause?

Indeed, you can in any case become pregnant. You might be less inclined to get pregnant during perimenopause, yet at the same it's as yet conceivable. However long you have a period, you can in any case get pregnant. To extend your family during this time, talk with your medical care supplier about your wellbeing, ripeness, and conceivable fruitfulness therapy choices.

At the point when your periods are unpredictable, you might be bound to get pregnant suddenly. To extend

your family at this age, keep utilizing anti-conception medication until your medical care supplier lets you know it's protected to stop. Keep on rehearsing safe sex to forestall physically sent contaminations (STIs) all through your life.

Living With

What inquiries would it be advisable for me to pose to my primary care physician?

Talk about your perimenopause side effects with your medical care supplier. It could assist with keeping a diary of your periods including when they start and stop and how much dying.

A few inquiries you ought to pose are:

Are these side effects of perimenopause?

How might I assuage my side effects?

How long do you figure I will have these side effects?

Could chemical treatment be a possibility for me?

Do I have to begin taking prescription or nutrients?

Are there any tests that ought to be finished?

Could I at any point actually become pregnant?

When would it be a good idea for me to call my primary care physician?

In the event that your perimenopausal side effects are horrendous or obstructing your personal satisfaction, it very well may be an ideal opportunity to contact your medical services supplier. They might have the option to offer help or prescribe a therapy to decrease the power of your side effects.

Will perimenopause influence my sexual coexistence?

Potentially. Certain side effects of perimenopause like vaginal dryness and uneasiness during sex can make having intercourse less alluring. Vaginal oils can be utilized to help dryness. Talk with your medical services supplier in the event that you dislike a diminished sex drive so they can prescribe ways of aiding you.

Would it be advisable for me to be on contraception during perimenopause?

Indeed. If you would rather not become pregnant, you ought to utilize conception prevention during perimenopause. Regardless of whether you are getting your period like clockwork, you are as yet ovulating during those months. Since it's impractical to foresee when you are ovulating, you ought to utilize contraception until you haven't gotten a period for something like a year.

Does perimenopause influence my rest?

Indeed, perimenopause can influence your rest. A few ladies in perimenopause experience a sleeping disorder and hindered rest because of night sweats or other menopausal side effects.

What do hot glimmers feel like during perimenopause?

A hot glimmer feels like an unexpected warmth all around your body. It is frequently joined by perspiring and a red, flushed face. Hot glimmers are brought about by low estrogen levels and can last months or years.

For what reason am I putting on weight during perimenopause?

The change in chemicals dials back your digestion. It's extremely normal for ladies in perimenopause to put on weight once their estrogen levels begin to decline. Keeping a solid eating routine and standard activity can assist with forestalling weight gain during the progress to menopause.

Note

Perimenopause is the change to menopause. During perimenopause, you might begin having menopause-like side effects, for example, hot glimmers, state of mind swings, or vaginal dryness. Most perimenopause side effects are sensible. In any case, on the off chance that you really want assistance overseeing side effects, prescriptions, and different medicines are accessible. Perimenopause closes when you've had no period for an entire year. By then, you enter menopause.

Conclusion

Menopause is something that all ladies should go through in the course of their lives. Thereare various kinds of menopause, various stages, various side effects, and different treatments.Each is subject to the ladies. There are different variables that influence a ladies' menopausalexperience and the ladies might need to make changes to their nourishment and exercise plans.